Every Man Who Looks in a Mirror

... sees a 16-year-old kid

And other middle-aged man reflections

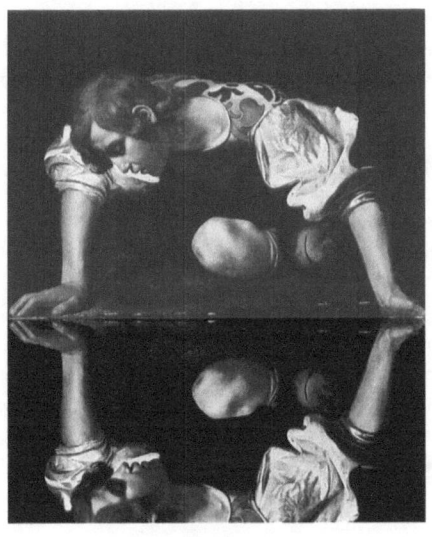

Edward Joseph Pierini, Jr.

Outskirts Press, Inc.

Denver, Colorado

Every Man Who Looks in a Mirror

. . . sees a 16-year-old kid

And other middle-aged man reflections

Outskirts Press, Inc.
http://www.outskirtspress.com
ISBN: 978-1-4787-2319-6

About the Cover

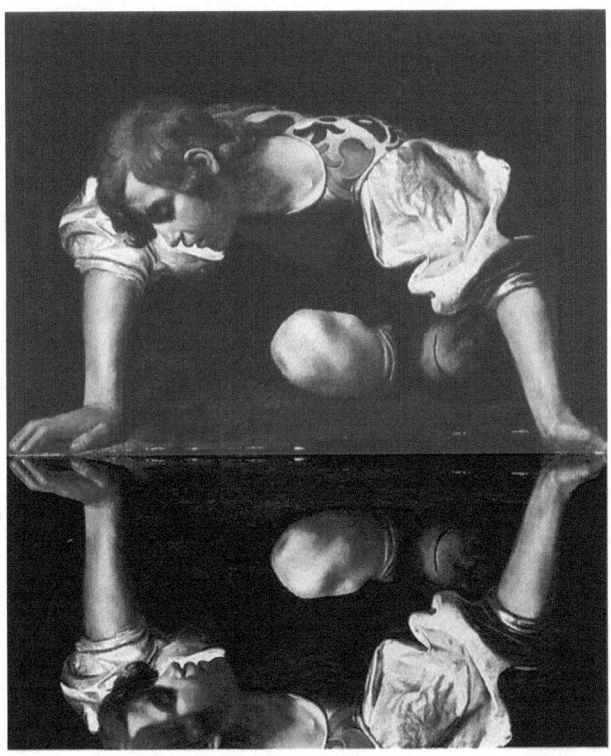

Narcissus is a painting by the great Italian artist Amerighi da Caravaggio who painted it circa 1597-1599. It's housed in the Galleria d'Arte Antica in Rome, Italy. The story of Narcissus, as told by Greek Mythology poet Ovid in his Metamorphoses, is of a handsome youth who falls in love with his own reflection, much like every man who looks in a mirror and sees a 16-year-old kid.

Dedication

I dedicate this book to my

Dad and Mom

They gave me life and much pleasure when seeing joy on their faces while reading my written reflections. My Dad and Mom have been my greatest fans. Rest in eternal peace my dear Dad.

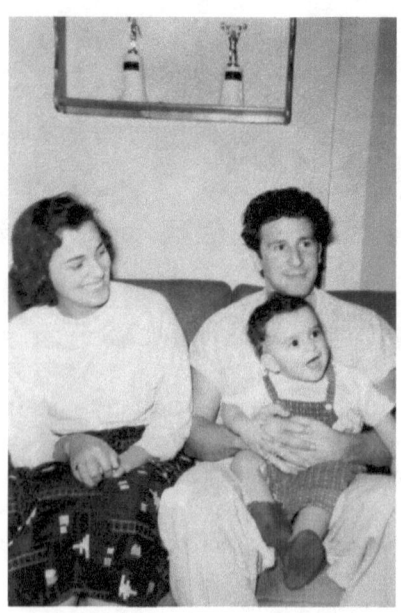

Acknowledgements

Thank You God, my Heavenly Father, for Your daily presence in my life.

Thank you my dear wife Elizabeth for your many comments and suggestions. They kept me honest and helped me express all my thoughts and feelings when writing this book.

Thank you my good friend Rick Sloan for your help designing this book cover. You did an excellent job creating the exact book cover I wanted.

I'll always be grateful to my dearly-departed maternal grandmother I knew as Gangee. Her special love contributed to my self-esteem that I first became aware of one day when looking at myself in a mirror. The rest is history and the title of my book.

Ed Pierin

Introduction

One day I realized I was a proud middle-aged man with thoughts and feelings about this and that meant to be shared with others.

This book is a collection of my 50 favorite middle-aged man written reflections expressing my thoughts and feelings about living and dying, gracefully aging, and trying my best to live a good and honest life.

Sharing these reflections is my modest attempt serving as an ambassador of middle-aged men around the world, advocating their interests and expressing their views about the way life was, the way life is and the way life should be.

Thanks for reading and have a wonderful life.

Ed Pierre

Content of Reflections

Every man who looks in a mirror sees a 16-year-old
kid 1-3
A middle-aged man...4-6
Except the 99- year- old man...................................7-8
The day before I die 9
Reading the obits...10-11
The fittest men resting in eternal peace 12-14
The day I conquered manual labor.......................15-17
Hiccups meant to be enjoyed 18-20
Greater than my own personal glory....................21-22
One of my first loves..23-25
Day 5 at my bachelor pad.....................................26-27
Taking good notes 28-30
Watching my teacher cry......................................31-33
I've been called it..34-36
Little white lies...37-39
If I should have done something different 40-41
I can, I shall and I will do.....................................42-43
What we had for breakfast....................................44-47
Holiday gluttony 48-50
From St. Thomas Aquinas......................................51-53
Zealously lethargic...54-55
Middle-aged man in motion 56-57
The day we went our separate way......................58-60
Until deaths do us part 61-63
Go away or here to stay?......................................64-66
Who am I to think I won't go first?.......................67-69
One day it will be our turn.................................... 70-71

Content of Reflections

Just the way we are 72

Who will be next? 76

Nothing I can do about it ....

Out of the loop 80

Sucker punched in a nightclub brawl....................... 83

Something is better than nothing............................. 86

Forever never made it back to the gym..................... 88

Give me a big head 90

For the rest of my life ....

In pursuit of gracefully aging 93

Diet and fitness affirmations from A to Z 96-1

Only 50 words... 1

Middle-aged man health and wellness exam 103-1

Like a splash of Old Spice...................................... 107-1

I miss my Gangee 110-1

Your son eternally... 1

Buona Pasqua 2013 113-1

Happy Birthday Dear Elizabeth............................... 115-1

Dime a dozen 117-1

My final 100 things 119-1

It was fun while it lasted....................................... 122-1

They're good and gone.. 125-1

Who are you? 129-1

A middle-aged man named Pierini 1

Note: These reflections are presented in no particular order. Select one to read each day according to your whim. After you've read it, put the book down and ponder what you've read for the rest of your day. Repeat each day for best results. Your mileage may vary.

Every man who looks in a mirror sees a 16-year-old kid

I've been looking at myself in a mirror for as long as I can remember. How many times who knows, but perhaps a number higher than I can count.

It's the honest truth if I'm rigorously honest. In fact, I enjoy it; not a little but a lot, and know I'm not alone among men.

I'm also sure the same is true for women but you'd have to ask a woman to be sure.

And based on my experiences, I've come to a conclusion that every man who looks in a mirror sees a 16-year-old kid; I do, or at least that's what I tell everyone.

And chances are so did the great Spanish explorer Ponce de Leon 500 years ago in his search for the fabled Fountain of Youth and a vision of eternal youth its discovery promised.

This daily visual exercise spares me of recognizing my obvious aging taking place daily because those changes are so subtle.

So much more pleasant to my eyes than visible changes I see in another person who I've not seen in a long time.

Like an old high school buddy I bump into who I haven't seen in 40 years. "Man did he get fat and old." I might say, or "Look at all his gray hair."

So how long can I get away with this?

A lot longer today than a generation ago because I can be like other men today and color my hair and moustache. It's much more common nowadays than the yesteryear grooming practices of my manly ancestors.

And I can have laser eye surgery helping me keep a youthful appearance rather than wearing eyeglasses making me look older.

I can even have liposuction ridding myself of any portly belly or excessive body fat I've grown. A century ago, these appendages were considered manly images of prosperity.

And thanks to modern day pharmacology and human growth hormone injections, I can now, along with other middle-aged men, have virility and explosiveness like a bottle of champagne repeatedly shook and waiting to be opened.

But despite these enhancements allowing me an illusion of being a 16-year-old kid, sooner or later Father Nature will catch up with me when a mirror can no longer lie.

Call it a fright of passage for lack of a better term; a realization I'm a middle-aged man at best or an old man in training.

But until that day comes, I'll continue having a great time when standing in front of a mirror washing my hands, shaving my beard, combing my hair, or brushing my teeth because every man who looks in a mirror sees a 16-year-old kid.

A middle-aged man

As the self-proclaimed ambassador of middle-aged men around the world, my first task is defining who's a middle-aged man.

By way of elimination, I'll start explaining who's an **old man**. Instructed by my Dad, he once shared how he had to get honest when turning age 70 by acknowledging he was now an old man. So an old man is anyone age 70 or older.

Old men are sometimes called senior citizens. I'm not an old man yet but hopefully one day I'll be one.

A **young man** becomes one at age 18; he's old enough to vote, eligible for military service, and may drink adult alcoholic beverages in many states. I was once a young man.

A young man remains one until age 45. "Why?" you ask; because I said so.

So what remains is a **middle-aged man**. This is someone between 45 and 70 years of age.

I'm a middle-aged man and have worn this badge of honor for more than a decade with, hopefully, many more years to go.

In the health and fitness world, as a middle-aged man, I'm only good as my last workout and I'm what I eat.

So I must train vigilantly and eat healthy, like a soldier preparing for combat duty. And, like a combat soldier, I do so out of fear and necessity.

Because in the darkness of night when caught off guard in a moment of weakness and with nobody looking, my middle-aged man body will scream it doesn't want to do it anymore - train and eat healthy.

Look at middle-aged men who've let themselves go by gaining excessive weight and becoming physically unfit.

Did they consciously make this decision one day when they were fit and healthy? I don't think so.

It creeps up with disguised and subtle temptation.

The temptation for them and me is how much more pleasant it is to come home after work, put on a pair of baggy worn green sweat pants with a loose drawstring, grab a bag of chips and flop on a comfortable and worn couch with television remote control in hand, and watch television shows nonstop until bedtime.

So training and eating healthy is something I must do. I know I'm only good as my last workout and I'm what I eat. Why? - Because, I'm a middle-aged man.

Except the 99-year-old man

For every middle-aged man I've talked to who told me they wouldn't want to live forever is one who wouldn't mind it.

Those who say they wouldn't may have witnessed an aging parent or relative suffering from a chronic or terminal illness.

They may have served as a caregiver witnessing the agony and pain of their loved one clinging to life at the very end.

My wife and I experienced this years ago when we brought an older person into our home. He had cancer and no immediate family to care for him.

We served as his comfort caregivers for a short time in the days leading up to his surgery. We witnessed his horrific agony and pain as cancer savagely attacked his body.

Despite his pain, this man had great hopes surgery would be successful so he could continue living. He preferred life rather than death.   God had a different plan for him, however, and he died about two months later.

I also witnessed this with my Dad who died an agonizing, painful and slow death from a rare cancer.   Despite witnessing my dear father withering away in horrific pain, he still wanted to live.

It's normal human behavior having this preference.   Even the most devoutly religious believing a wonderful eternal life awaits them in heaven generally prefer a little more time on planet earth. So I guess this means I'm normal.

With this preference of life rather than death, I have thoughts of old being what other people are, and I'm only old if there's not someone who's older than me. So this means I'm not old.

An elderly friend who was 89-years-young at the time once said it best when he told me "Ain't no man wants to live to be 100 except the 99-year-old man."

The day before I die

I once read a touching news article about a retired schoolteacher who had a lifelong dream of completing her bachelor's degree in education.

She reached her milestone nearly three weeks after her 100th birthday and then died the following day.

I've privately thought and shared before that no man wants to live to be 100 except the 99-year-old man.

Reading about this retired schoolteacher's accomplishment makes me realize some of what I hope to achieve in my life may not be accomplished until the day before I die.

Reading the obits

It's a daily ritual for most middle-aged men, including me, of reading newspaper obituaries (obits) and funeral notices.

As a native of the city whose daily newspaper I read, frequently I learn of a former school classmate, long-lost acquaintance, client or friend departing planet earth for greener pastures.

I read obits and funeral notices each morning scanning them in a flurry like how my wife shops for a dress at a bargain department store.

Except she moves dresses quickly from left to right on the rack from which they hang while I scan obits and funeral notices in alphabetical order from top to bottom.

Just like my wife, I'm looking for a find. Her find is a great bargain while my find is a name of someone I know or knew. Like her, sometimes I come up empty and other times I make a find.

Reading obits and funeral notices is something I like to do. It takes me down memory lane to a time when life seemed simpler and more youthful.

But it's also an eerie reminder of with each breath I take is one less breath left in my life. It gives me a reality check of one day I'll get my turn just like the person whose obit or funeral notice I've read.

And that's good because it keeps me honest by not taking my life for granted or the lives of anyone else.

It makes me want to be the best I can today, tomorrow, and each and every day remaining in my life.

It does me so much good that I'll continue reading the obits.

The fittest men resting in eternal peace

One sunny and tranquil Sunday afternoon, my wife and I visited the oldest officially established graveyards in Sacramento, the Sacramento City Cemetery.

It's a resting place for more than 25,000 pioneers, immigrants, and their families and descendents.

Among those calling it home are city founder Captain John A. Sutter, Jr. and other big shots from Sacramento's early years.

Thousands of early settlers are buried here representing the historical and cultural diversity of Sacramento with many symbolic monuments of Victorian-era funeral customs.

Many old graves are those of babies and young children who died in floods. There were many floods in early Sacramento before the entire city was raised in order to escape river flooding.

People also died from fires during some of these floods and, they too, are buried here.

Visiting cemeteries fascinates me; I've visited many in cities and countries around the world.

My calculating-thirsty mind always wants to use information etched on a grave marker to calculate how old a person was when they passed away.

In a reflective moment, I ponder how someday someone will look at my grave marker and calculate how long I lived.

While people then did not live as long as we now do, some nonetheless lived very long lives. This always makes me wonder about their secrets to their long lives.

Our visit was a very relaxing couple hours on a beautiful Sunday afternoon with pleasant sunshine providing a welcoming reminder of a spring season about to begin.

Flowers were blossoming and birds were chirping a melody so pleasant to my ears, mind and spirit.

As our stay ended, thoughts entered my mind of coming back soon for another visit. I also briefly pondered the day of my one-way trip to the cemetery of my final resting place.

Until this day comes, I'll continue chasing good fitness and health preparing me to be among the fittest men resting in eternal peace.

The day I conquered manual labor

Those who embrace it generally figure it out early in life while those who fight it may never.

What I'm talking about is work as in my job or career. It consumes at least one-third of my adult life.

My first job was picking tomatoes but that was more a youthful cultural experience than a real job.

If the amount of money I made from this short work experience was lard, I never made enough to grease a frying pan.

My next pre-teenager job was helping my Dad when he owned a commercial janitorial business. Later, as a teenager, I worked in a factory and restaurants.

I purchased an electric guitar with earnings from my janitor assistant job. The factory job is how I bought my first car. The restaurant jobs gave me money to buy gasoline for my car and extra teenager spending change.

None of these work experiences adequately prepared me for what was to follow as a soldier in the U.S. Army. For the next three years, I experienced a Monday through Friday day in and day out "manual labor" grind.

Even though I had an easy military job working in a personnel office, this work was my introduction to a force within me of resisting manual labor. It provided me many valuable lessons about the role of work in my life.

And what's this role?

It's that work is a natural part of a balanced and healthy life, just like breathing, eating, exercising, praying, sleeping, and socializing.

It should be enjoyable. If it's not, then something isn't right needing to be fixed to achieve balance and harmony in my life.

So whether I'm a big shot CEO of a Fortune 500 company, a high-priced attorney making big money chasing ambulances, a hospital emergency room physician saving lives, a gardener raking leaves, a manual laborer digging ditches, or an unpaid volunteer doing charitable works, it's all the same in that, like them, I grind away doing my thing bringing home the bacon.

At times it feels demanding as manual labor. It exhausts me making me want to run away. Work is a never-ending perpetual challenge of accepting and embracing it as a necessary part my life.

I believe it takes at least 10 years conquering these demons and embracing work as something good for me.

I remember when I did – the day I conquered manual labor.

Hiccups meant to be enjoyed

Today is the first Saturday of the year I'm working. I always start working half days on Saturday beginning in February. It's the start of my busy work season lasting until April.

What I've discovered over many years of doing this are the different seasons of my relationship with work.

Starting a new year, I slowly begin awakening for an upcoming busy work season waiting for me. I'm much like a bear awakening from winter hibernation.

My work productivity erosion is at its peak from an extended slack season. I'm very much like an old stiff rodeo cowboy who has fallen off a bucking bronco one time too many. I move ever so slowly going from here to there while I work.

Once awakened, I begin conquering my work productivity erosion. I slowly rid myself of sleep in my work ethic.

Slowly but surely, I start working harder and longer much like a migrant farm laborer picking fruit when crops are in season.

There's really no big deal about my hard work when thinking about it in a yesteryear context of my ancestors working hard every day while chasing their dreams in their new country.

March is normally my hardest month because I'll work about 250 hours. April is more of the same for half the month.

Then my busy work season screeches to a halt. I echo long and loud mental and physical sighs of relief.

At this point, it's not uncommon for me to experience a serious adrenaline hangover or have feelings like a victim of abuse from the constant demands to which my body, mind and spirit have been subjected.

Then a fun season begins with my very relaxed work schedule. When all goes well, I work Tuesday through Thursday from 9:00 a.m. to 3:00 p.m. during this fun season.

It's wonderful this time of the year with only occasional departures from my leisure schedule to meet special client demands.

Sure it's possible for me to accept additional clients, work harder and make more money, but why is the question I ask myself when these thoughts enter my head.

My answer is always the same because my wealth of leisure is golden.

It's during this leisure season my work productivity erosion slowly returns to former levels where it again takes all day for me to get nothing done.

It's the flip side of Parkinson's Law – the classic economic adage of *"Work expands for the time available to complete it."* – in that my leisure time at work expands for the time I have to be leisurely.

The lesson I've learned from these seasons of my work is that, just like winter, spring, summer and fall, work seasons come and go just like hiccups meant to be enjoyed.

Greater than my own personal glory

Many times I've had an opportunity of giving advice to others facing a challenging activity or event in their lives.

There's one tip I give them before undertaking their challenge, whether it's something related to career, family, fitness, health or relationships.

This tip is something I've also followed in my own challenges. I personally discovered it many years ago when my son ran cross country in high school.

At a meet one day, I suggested he offer up his race effort for Jason's father, one of my former karate buddies who recently died too early in his life from a heart attack.

My son and I both knew Jason and his father, and we both felt sad about Jason losing his father.

Well my son ran a good race that day. I'm sure offering his race performance for the memory of Jason's father gave it meaning and purpose.

My son's good race day performance that day was for something greater than his own personal glory.

It's the same for me. By offering a challenging effort for something more than my own personal glory, I add meaning and purpose to my effort that's greater than my own personal glory.

If I'm successful, then I also have my glory like frosting on a cake.

This offering gives me comfort and support of not being alone in those dark and lonely moments of a big challenge.

I experience true joy when offering my challenging efforts for something greater than my own personal glory.

One of my first loves

One of my first loves was "born" in 1963 when I was an 8–year-young boy in 3rd grade, when thousands of Americans were driving their 1963 Pontiac Grand Prix automobiles.

Eight years later in 1971, one would be my first car.

It all began in the summer of 1970 with a part-time summer job working at the Duncan Hines Division of Proctor & Gamble, dumping 100-pound sacks of flour into bins used to produce cake mix.

I made $2.00 an hour working Monday through Friday from 7:30 a.m. to 11:30 a.m. and felt like a "rich man" because minimum wage was only $1.65 an hour in those days.

I earned $40.00 a week before taxes were deducted. My weekly paycheck was $36.41 and payday was every Friday.

My Mom drove me to and from work every day. Every Friday on the way home, we stopped at the bank where I deposited

$30.00 of my paycheck into a savings account. I kept the remaining $6.41 for weekly spending money.

I did this every week that summer and eventually, with some other savings, had enough money to buy my first car - a red 1963 Pontiac Grand Prix with a white vinyl top.

It cost a whopping $475 and buying it drained my savings account.

Every middle-aged man remembers his first car and I'm no exception. It was a gas-guzzler averaging about 9 miles a gallon, so many of my memories of it are being at a gas station filling up an empty gas tank.

Gasoline then was about 30-35 cents a gallon so a full tank cost about $6.00 and lasted an entire week.

My other memories include driving to and from school every day, going to the drive-in movies with friends, cruising around the neighborhood with the radio blasting, and washing and waxing my car every week.

I never took a photo of this car so my pleasant yesteryear memories of it are those in my mind's eye.

As a middle-aged man, every time I look in a mirror I see a 16-year-old kid, and when I think of being a 16-year-old kid, I fondly remember my 1963 Pontiac Grand Prix, one of my first loves.

Day five at my bachelor pad

Today is another day at my bachelor pad. I've been alone ever since my wife left five days ago to attend a one-week retreat in another state and then spend a few more days visiting our son who lives there.

She's about 650 miles away from home right now enjoying her retreat, warmer weather, and a time-out from me and all my middle-aged man callousness, grouchiness and hardness.

All alone, my life has been business as usual these past five days because I'm a middle-aged man creature of habit.

My daily ritual is a script so predictable I can do it blindfolded and set my watch to it.

But in a pause from my routine life, thoughts creep into my head of what I could do differently during my silent retreat, or "wife-fast" for lack of a better description.

The mischief I could find, the no good I could do, the late nights I could frequent, and wee hours of the morning I could witness and determine they still exist.

I could return home just in time at the crack of dawn resuming my routine life and then repeat this mischief again later the same night.

Nobody would know. It would be my little secret if I played my cards right.

Yes, nobody would know except me.

But as tempting as it seems I'll skip this mischief and stay close to home because I'm a middle-aged man, and a devoted and faithful husband of 35 years. I've got battle scars to prove it.

I'm very content staying close to home living day five at my bachelor pad.

Taking good notes

With paper and pencil in hand, I remember taking notes in elementary school as my teacher stood in front of the classroom chalkboard teaching her students.

I didn't take as many notes during my middle and high school years because, sadly, academics weren't a priority for me.

In college, however, I was a motivated student thanks to earlier lessons learned as a U.S. Army soldier about the importance of getting a good formal education.

Once again, with paper and pencil in hand, I took good notes of everything my college professors uttered in their lectures.

I've always been blessed with a good memory and attention to detail so, good notes along with diligent study served me well. I got good grades on all my exams and quizzes.

Well almost four decades later, I find myself taking notes again, this time when observing or listening to my elders because there's so much to learn from them.

Insights they provide about the life they've lived and want to live are too important for this good student to miss.

I take notes of their thoughts about living and dying in their now golden years, how they handle difficult situations, if and how they exercise, and the relative importance of faith, family, fitness, fortune and health in their lives.

What they tell me is as fascinating and instructive as a college philosophy professor's lecture on ethics almost 40 years ago, and as thought-provoking as a sermon on redemptive suffering given by a priest during a Sunday Mass homily.

Every now and then, I'm blessed with an opportunity of talking to someone who's 90-years-young or older.

I always reach for a pen and paper during these golden opportunities realizing what a treasure it is being in their company taking notes.

In a moment of reflection, I imagine what it'll be like one day when someone else is taking notes of what they see in me and words of wisdom I'll hopefully share.

Maybe it's already happening and, in my aloofness, I haven't a clue.

At this point in my life, I know more today than yesterday but less than tomorrow.

There's so much more to know and learn and I'll do so by taking good notes.

Watching my teacher cry

Ask older people what they were doing when learning of President John F. Kennedy's assassination on November 22, 1963 and chances are they'll have a quick answer for you.

I was a third grade student on the school playground during recess when learning the news.

After recess, I remember sitting in my classroom desk watching my teacher cry while she told us President Kennedy had been assassinated.

It was awkward watching an adult cry but now I better understand because, as a middle-aged man, I've shed my own adult tears.

Later in the evening at home, I remember watching non-stop television coverage of this terrible moment in American history on our black and white television set.

Every television station provided nonstop coverage of this tragic event. Regular television programs were cancelled for several days.

This was a time in my boyhood life when every Saturday morning I would wake up early and watch the Original Superman show on television.

I remember being anxious Friday night thinking Superman might not be television the following morning. Superman was very high on my priority list in those days.

I also remember waking up early the next morning and being disappointed when the show didn't air as normally scheduled.

In its place was television news coverage giving me lasting and vivid memories of President Kennedy's casket covered with an American flag.

Superman continued to be on my mind while television news coverage continued hour after hour with no break for commercials.

I now realize my young boy behavior showed a youthful misguided sense of priorities in the context of this national tragedy. My behavior was inexcusable.

It makes me reflect about how I'm still predisposed to similar misguided priorities, except now I can't blame it on being a boy.

So I tell myself there's more growing up for me to do even as a middle-aged man.

Every November 22nd I like to pause and say a private prayer for the departed soul of President John F. Kennedy, wondering if he's in Heaven looking down on our great nation that entrusted him with the highest honor of serving his country as President.

I'll always remember November 22, 1963, the day President John F. Kennedy was assassinated, sitting in my classroom desk watching my teacher cry.

I've been called it

Thus far in my life journey, I've worn many hats and have had many friendships and relationships.

Closer to home, I am and have been a husband, father, son, grandson, great-grandson, brother, brother-in-law, nephew, cousin, and uncle.

Outside of family and home, I am and have been a classmate, college student, friend, soldier, veteran, karateka, fitness buff or dude, and co-worker to name a few.

Closer to self, I've called myself the ambassador of middle-aged men around the world. Being an ambassador is serious business and I wear this badge of honor with upmost responsibility.

This list is not all-inclusive but rather than add to it, I'll stop while I'm ahead because I might forget where I'm going with this reflection.

And where am I going? I'm glad you asked.

It was to list some of the adjectives and other descriptive expressions I've been called by others.

Some are good and others aren't so good. I'm grateful to have been called the good ones while the bad ones I could do without.

What are some of the bad ones?

I've been called a jerk for starters. I've also been described as bad, dumb, mean, cruel, and callous to name a few.

Want me to name more?

How about aloof, selfish, narcissistic, devious, evil, show-off, stupid and insensitive?

I could go on and on but it's not necessary because I see the picture of this unpleasant character others have accurately painted of me.

If movie ratings were used to rate names and expressions I've been called, I'd be an owner of a few G ratings and many R-ratings and X-ratings.

For every day there's a night, for every action there's a reaction, for every push there's a pull, for every positive there's a negative, for every yin there's a yang, and so on.

That's certainly true with what people have and do say about me. I'm the good, the bad and the ugly all in one.

While being on the receiving end of these unfavorable descriptions, I've always had a quick response saying how I'd be worried if the only thing people had to say about me were good things.

What's that all about?

Is it another instance of another character defect rather than me acknowledging there's something about me needing work?

This is something I must further reflect on in my life journey of being the best I can so let me close by saying if you can think of it, I've been called it.

Little white lies

As a kid growing up I remember the phrase "Liar liar pants on fire!" yelled when catching another kid telling a lie.

Telling lies, mostly little white lies, was a regular and necessary evil, and an adolescent survival tool.

Telling little white lies was not just a kid thing for me because I've told my fair share as an adult. As a middle-aged man, I still struggle with a temptation of wanting to tell them.

So what's a **lie** and how does it differ from a **little white lie**. Here's what I've read.

A **lie** is a deceptive untruthful statement told solely for the purpose of deceiving someone else. It may involve maintaining a secret or reputation, protecting someone's feelings, or avoiding getting caught doing something wrong and the punishment that comes along with it.

A **white lie** is a less serious lie. It may have different meanings in different cultures but, in general, is told to avoid harmful realistic implications of the truth.   Many consider little white lies to be harmless.

That makes me a liar and a little white liar. My friends on the school playground were right!

So a little angel sits on my right shoulder telling me I'm lying or telling me I shouldn't because it's not right.   On my other shoulder sits a little devil telling me it's OK because it's just a little white lie.

I'm lying when I tell a client his work was not completed on time because of computer problems when the real reason was my procrastination.

This reflection seems so trivial in context of a bigger picture, such as when Presidential candidates and politicians tell us little white lies. If it's not wrong for them then how can it be wrong for me?

It's wrong for me because, as a middle-aged man, I've discovered the virtue of rigorous honesty.

Whether or not rigorous honesty is good for them has no bearing of it being good for me.

At this point in my life, I'm trying my best being rigorously honest with everyone, including myself.

It's the right thing to do as difficult as it may be so I'll continue struggling to do so in my truthful rest-of-life journey.

At this point in my life, I'm trying my best to not tell any little white lies.

If I should have done something different

I've previously shared it's a daily ritual for most middle-aged and elderly people to read newspaper obituaries and funeral notices.

One morning while reading mine, I learned a longtime client died at a too young age of 51 years.

In recent years, I hadn't had frequent face-to-face meetings with him because we'd do business by mail and telephone.

Months before his death, however, he visited me bringing some documents needed for work I was doing for him. His visit gave both of us an opportunity to chat and catch up on how we've been doing.

While engaging in our middle-aged man small talk, I looked deep into his eyes and saw a person who had aged a lot and did not appear healthy. I also smelled a strong scent of alcohol on his breath.

It was a sad sight leaving me feeling unsure about what to say or do so I did nothing remaining silent.

The rest of our brief and unscheduled meeting was more middle-aged man small talk including a "How's your boy doing?" question from me. He loved his 14-year-old son with all his heart.

That was the last time I saw him.

I'll never ask and probably never know why his life ended so soon at a too young age of 51 years and, honestly, it's really none of my business.

After I read his obituary, I reflected about the last time I saw him while quietly asking myself if I should have done something different.

I can, I shall, and I will do

They're a dime a dozen, those "could-a, should-a and would-a" people who find comfort in their misery spending excessive time thinking and talking about what they could have, should have or would have done in their past.

Sometimes I also sit in a pity pot engaging in my own negative self-talk.

There's nothing wrong taking a lesson from failure chapters from my book of life, particularly if doing so helps me develop success-oriented action plans for my future.

I shouldn't, however, excessively dwell there stuck in my stinking thinking like a pickup truck stuck in mud in the middle of a farm orchard after a winter storm.

It serves no moving-forward benevolent purpose other than keeping me stuck in my historical failure and misery.

It's a misery that, if I allow it, radiates and burns within my psyche and soul. It may also be within auditory reach of others looking to me for comfort, inspiration and wisdom with challenges in their own lives.

It's like me shouting, "Hey I feel like crap and want to bring you down with me!"

Sometimes I have to let this downward spiraling stinking thinking run its course to where I just get sick and tired of being sick and tired.

Sooner or later, hitting my negative thinking rock bottom, realizing it and then looking upward at a blue sky, I acknowledge wanting something better for myself.

Join me right now for each remaining breath of life and let's together chant an empowering affirmation of "I can, I shall and I will do."

What we had for breakfast

It's a frequent daily occurrence like my morning shave; a moment of middle-aged man memory fog or, as a friend calls it, a case of **CRS** or "can't remember stuff."

It goes with the turf at this stage of my life, and knowing I'm not alone comforts me.

I also feel comforted when witnessing younger people go blank in their mental memory department but know their reasons for memory fog are different than mine.

I'm aware of differences between short-term and long-term memory loss. The former is what periodically afflicts me while the latter is a problem for others.

The short-term stuff can be further classified into other non-scientific categories.

There's selective forgetfulness my wife reminds me I have when it comes to things I've promised to do or not do again.

She reminds me I don't have a memory problem because I always remember to do things I enjoy. How true this is.

Then there's aloofness, absent-mindedness or carelessness; these seem to be different than true memory loss.

Take my wife for example. She frequently "loses" her cell phone or car keys but I don't believe she has a memory loss problem.

The truth is she seldom loses anything and neither do we. It's better said we merely forget where we've placed our lost items.

Why do I find joy witnessing another middle-aged man or woman whose mind and memory have temporarily gone blank?

Maybe it's a hilarious and joyful laughter I get from looking at a blank look on their faces triggering endorphins in my mind, much like a runner who experiences a runner's high.

Or maybe it's because I get momentary relief from my own memory-lapse misery while finding delight in another's plight.

Yet in the same breath, I always rise to the occasion of helping my memory loss-stricken comrades, guiding them safely out of whatever deep memory fog they're experiencing.

These moments are acts of charity. They're like a father coaching his son taking a first ride on a training wheels-free shiny red bicycle.

My *"You can do it!"* comforting facial expressions while looking into their eyes provide emotional food for their souls.

During their bouts, I remain ever so patient with them as if listening to someone stuttering while speaking.

These moments make me realize I'm like them because it happens to me too except now it's their turn and mine will come later.

Eventually, we come out of a dark bottom forgetfulness abyss and are able to complete our thoughts that, moments earlier, had temporarily vanished in bright daylight.

As they or I bask in glory of being able to pull it off once again, I always conclude this bonding experience we just shared with a comment always bringing a laugh.

I tell them – or myself - all is well if we can remember what we had for breakfast.

Holiday gluttony

A dictionary defines gluttony as an act or habit of eating to excess. Gluttony is an unregulated love for food and drink.

It's been around as long as man and his food and drink. The great philosopher St. Augustine wrote about gluttony in his classic book *The Confessions of St. Augustine*.

He shared it's an appetite out of control causing him to abuse healthy pleasures God has given to eating and drinking.

Gluttony makes me behave like an animal although I'm not sure animals overeat or drink as much as I sometimes do.

My holiday gluttony season normally lasts 36 days beginning Thanksgiving Day and ending after New Year's Day.

The challenge I face with my gluttony cross is not much different than what St. Augustine experienced over one thousand six hundred years ago.

St. Augustine wrote that by eating and drinking we repair daily decays of our body.

This necessity of eating and drinking was sweet to him, but he fought not to be taken captive by it.

Hunger and thirst were his pains and, like a fever, they burned until aided by the medicine of nourishment necessary for good health.

He wrote:

> *Thus, whereas health is the cause of eating and drinking, yet a dangerous delight accompanies those activities and for the most part endeavors to take precedence so that I may do for its sake what I pretend and desire to do for health's sake.*

St. Augustine shared he was uncertain whether it was the necessary care of his body asking for sustenance or the voluptuous deceit of greediness that proffered its services.

My 21st-century challenges with gluttony are similar to those experienced by St. Augustine in the fourth century.

How often will I eat during this holiday season because food and drink are abundantly available rather than because I'm really hungry or thirsty?

Is it really physical hunger or thirst I'm experiencing or something deeper residing in my spirit, never to be satisfied by any amount of food and drink?

These are questions I ask myself while standing on guard from my own predispositions to holiday gluttony.

From St. Thomas Aquinas

The number of people in America suffering from mental disorders grows by leaps and bounds as new mental disorders are discovered and named.

Those characters known as psychiatrists and psychologists have discovered a new one.

Experts have stated there's now enough evidence to call binge eating a mental disorder.

It's defined as eating large amounts of food when you're not hungry and then feeling disgusted and depressed afterwards.

According to one psychiatrist, there's no consensus as to what's the best treatment for someone afflicted with a binge eating mental disorder.

He added, however, several types of medications appear helpful. I'm sure his comment is pleasant music to the ears of the pharmaceutical industry.

Well I've got some good news for these characters – they're a day late and a dollar short with their new finding.

This disorder shouldn't be called binge eating because it's really gluttony.

Gluttony is gulping down or swallowing – as in over-indulgence and over-consumption – food, drink or intoxicants to a point of waste.

In some Christian denominations, gluttony is considered one of the seven deadly sins.

St. Thomas Aquinas, a great and immensely influential philosopher and Catholic theologian, classified six ways in which gluttony is committed:

Praepropere – eating too soon

Laute – eating too expensively

Nimis – eating too much

Ardenter – eating too eagerly

Studiose – eating too daintily

Forente – eating wildly

If I ever one day suffer from binge eating and reach out for help and answers, I'll not buy the latest self-help book for guidance.

I know better answers and guidance are available from St. Thomas Aquinas.

Zealously lethargic

After a conversation with someone, I'll often wish them good faith, family, fitness, fortune and health.

It's one of my expressions in the same category as "Have a good day!" and other blindly-expressed and robotic utterances sounding more cliché than "See you later." or "Good-bye."

What exactly does it mean to others and me when I say to have good faith, family, fitness, fortune and health?

How do I measure qualities of these attributes?

How do I go about my daily life pursuing them?

Do I do so deliberately with focus, or haphazardly without clarity?

And finally, how bad do I want good faith, family, fitness, fortune and health?

Do I want it only if served on a silver platter, or do I want it bad enough to eat, breathe and sleep it in my day-to-day activities?

By golly, I want it but wonder and doubt if I'm always willing to do the hard work required.

Whenever setting goals and resolutions, I reflect on how I'm doing in pursuing good faith, family, fitness, fortune and health.

Am I doing so with youthful passion and purpose or like a middle-aged man who's zealously lethargic?

Middle-aged man in motion

One day while buying a cup of coffee, I asked the person taking my order if she was a track athlete in high school. I privately guessed she was about my age.

She replied yes to my question and was curious why I asked.

I explained how athletic-like and quickly she moved from the cash register to another area behind the counter when filling my order.

Driving to work, I thought about what people see when watching me in motion.

Do I move like an athlete with explosive take off speed and a brisk pace when walking or taking a flight of stairs?

Or do I move like a lethargic middle-aged man strolling at a snail's pace with hands in my pockets whistling Dixie?

Do I stand tall with a strong lower back arch, expanded chest, an upright upper body, and a strong rooted stance capable of lifting a heavy load?

Or, do I have a forward lean accompanied by a frail look of ready to collapse if a heavy object was placed in my carrying arms?

What's my truth when in motion has been a question ringing in my mind since that morning observation.

As a middle-aged man, it's easy for me to lack rigorous honesty in assessments of my physical self.

What about you? Join me thinking about what people see when looking at this middle-aged man in motion.

The day we went our separate way

The exact day escapes me but I'm guessing it was almost ten years ago. Who would have thought we wouldn't spend our entire life together. We'd been together so long.

I remember my first glance so ever long ago, knowing it was love at first sight. We spent countless hours together every morning, day and night.

As our relationship grew, I remember our time spent together increased to a point where it became more important than other things I could or should be doing.

As is often the case in all relationships, however, there came a point when I took things for granted. I became complacent, and soon found I wasn't excited in our relationship like before.

I became less aroused with my partner, eventually having episodes of performance anxiety, and finding it increasing difficult to do it.

Intimacy started to fade and before long I became interested, again, in going to places where I hadn't been in a long time. I now wanted to do things with different people.

This continued for a while until it was time for me to get honest and break the news that our relationship was over.

We could still remain friends and cherish good times spent together, but that inseparable relationship bonded by a deep love for each other was now a thing of our past.

As is the case in all broken relationships, I had initial hurt and felt lonely especially at night.

Holidays and special occasions were tough for me because of so many pleasant memories I had of good times we spent together.

But by reaching out to others, and responding to invitations to go here and do this and that, new healthy activities and relationships started to be part of my life.

Once again, my life now had meaning, purpose and zeal. I again felt in love and loved.

Every now and then I look back and remember the family television I gave away, and the day we went our separate way.

Until deaths do us part

One evening during a small family gathering for my 54th birthday, before the barbeque ribs, steak, salad and dessert were served, I went to a funeral rosary for a man our family knew fifty years earlier.

His family and our family were neighbors and friends until we moved to a different city and lost contact with them.

Eduardo A. had recently died after 92 years of life. I learned of his passing while reading newspaper obituaries, one of my favorite middle-aged man daily rituals.

Upon learning of his passing, I had a strong desire wanting to attend his rosary service and decided I would. I invited my Mom and she joined me.

As is often the case when attending funerals, I did so out of respect but also to satisfy my own curiosity.

Would I recognize Mr. A. resting in peace in his open casket? Would I recognize his wife and two sons?

Would they recognize my Mom and me and have memories of my family like we had of them? Fifty years ago is a long time I thought to myself.

As we prayed the Holy Rosary, I learned Mr. A. was a man believing in God and his Catholic faith because the rosary is definitely a Catholic form of prayer.

Afterwards, various acquaintances and family members gave brief accounts of their Mr. A. memories followed by a short photo slide show of him at various stages of his long life.

I watched and listened attentively yearning to know more about him and the long life he lived.

There were many clues about what he valued most: his faith, his family and his moustache.

Other than a couple old black and white photos of him as a young boy, every other photo showed a proud family man with an ever-present and groomed moustache.

After his service ended, I approached his open casket paying my final respects. I noticed his groomed white moustache as he lay so ever peaceful in eternal rest.

I like attending funerals because they remind me how precious life is, and how my time on earth is limited and at the pleasure of God.

They also remind me that, despite all I do for my fitness and health, one day my life will come to an end just like Mr. A.

Funerals also give me an opportunity of being grateful for the most important things in life. It's not the money I make, economic wealth I amass, big shots I know or places visited in my travels.

It's much simpler than that as Mr. A. reminded me. I discovered both what he did and I do value the most - our faith, our family and our moustache – until deaths do us part.

Go away or here to stay?

"Gray, gray go away and come back another day!"

Daily early morning meetings with my bathroom mirror are revealing new gray hair on my head and white moustache whiskers below my nose.

They're constant and nagging reminders from Father Nature that I'm a middle-aged man in full blossom and an old man in training.

What should this middle-aged man do?

Unlike middle-aged men from yesteryear, many from my generation have borrowed a solution middle-aged women have been using for years – coloring or highlighting their gray wisdom streaks.

To be or not to be is my dilemma and question. Should I continue being a gray-haired middle-aged man?

Exploring my options, I visited an internet website selling hair products for graying men wanting to do something about it, or stay in the game as the website describes.

Maybe staying in the game is what I want to do.

I learned this company offers two solutions. The first one gets rid of all my gray hair in five minutes while the second one allows me to keep a little gray.

I can buy either product online and the good news is the first order is completely free.

There's no mention if they ship their product in a plain brown box with no outward clue it's a hair coloring product.

That's very important to me, I reflected, because this gray-haired middle-aged man likes his privacy about vanity matters like this.

As an alternative to buying their product online, I could travel to a distant city wearing a pair of dark sunglasses and buy it at a store. I could pay for it with cash not leaving any clues or evidence of my purchase.

I could protect my privacy and keep this a closely-guarded secret. Nobody would know but me.

After much deliberation in solitude, I've chosen to keep my gray hair and white whiskers instead of joining other middle-aged men who've chosen to juice their hair with an infinite selection of colors under the rainbow.

I've decided there's more than one way to stay in the game. That's my decision today but tomorrow may be different.

Every morning when looking in a mirror, I can choose to admire my gray hair and white whiskers or be in agony about them while asking myself, "Go away or here to stay?"

Who am I to think I won't go first?

Yesterday I took a different route to visit my Dad on Father's Day. I drove past a cemetery where many of my relatives are resting in eternal peace.

One day I'll join them because my wife, in her "plan for the future and leave no stone unturned" determination, purchased our gravesites there several years ago.

The cemetery was crowded with cars and people making their annual Father's Day visit placing flowers on gravesites, saying a few prayers, and fondly remembering good old days with their fathers.

I'm an odd-ball who likes visiting cemeteries and strolling up and down rows of gravesites reading the name, date of birth, date of death and anything else engraved on grave markers.

Being numerically-oriented, I quickly calculate how old a person was when they passed away while wondering who they were and the life they lived.

I'm fascinated when discovering someone who lived a long time ago and a very long life. I wonder about their secret to their long life.

About 10 minutes after passing the cemetery, I arrived at my Dad's house. We had a nice time together and great conversation about his good old days.

How many more Father's Days my Dad will have is my "anyone's guess" reflection.

If I had it my way, I'd like at least a dozen more.

The truth is, a reflective thought reminds me, one day he'll get called home for his eternal rest.

When this day comes, those Father's Day trips visiting him will be to the cemetery I drove past while traveling to his house.

But there are no guarantees in life. Maybe that's not how it'll turn out because, "Who am I to think I won't go first?

Post-script: My father passed away on May 24, 2013. He did go first. I visited his grave about one month later on Father's Day 2013.

Rest in eternal peace my dear Dad.

One day it will be our turn

Sooner or later most middle-aged men and women will face the elder-care needs of their aging parents.

People are living longer than before and so are our mothers and fathers.

The challenges we face may be formidable because elderly and needy parents oftentimes don't reveal their needs. In true parent fashion, they don't want to burden their children.

They may also be in denial they're reaching a point in their elder lives of needing extra help.

It can be an emotional and tough situation for adult children of elderly and needy parents, particularly if they live far away in another city or state.

It was very tough watching my father age and die while he replied all was well and he didn't need any help in response to my inquiries and offers.

There comes a time when taking care of Mom and Dad takes precedence over the fun things we'd rather be doing with what little spare time we have.

There's nothing more honorable than rising to the occasion of being a good son or daughter to our elderly parents in need, fully aware that, like Mom and Dad, one day it will be our turn.

Just the way we are

What's a healthy body image? Do I have one or might I have a body image disorder?

These are tough questions requiring rigorous honesty if I'm to get truthful answers buried deep in my middle-aged man mind closely guarded by a fortress of denial.

It's easy for me to blame the media for any body image disorders I may have because they often promote unrealistic ones of men and women.

But doing so doesn't address any underlying reasons having their origin in something more significant than television programs I view or advertisement I read.

In one of my earlier reflections, and the title of this book, I wrote that every man who looks in a mirror sees a 16-year-old kid.

If I took myself seriously, this would definitely be a king size example of a serious body image disorder.

What about something a little more real and serious?

I once had an e-mail exchange with a young man fitness acquaintance who shared he may have a body image disorder.

He's a fit and strong person with a physique reflecting the training dues he has paid. He's at the tail end of young manhood and a couple years away from entering a great period of middle-aged manhood.

In an e-mail exchange, he shared the following with me:

> *I have an unhealthy image of my body. I am constantly evaluating and JUDGING how I look or worry how I will be perceived by others. In fact, when I look in the mirror I still see a 16 year old skinny kid who desperately is trying to get bigger.*
>
> *That's the inner child in me screaming for acceptance and positive feedback; something obviously I really didn't get growing up and now it has surfaced in my body image.*
>
> *In my desperate attempts to gain weight, I remember downing gallons of whole milk and chocolate chip cookies daily.*

The tighter my shirts or jeans felt the better I felt about myself. The power of feeling "big" gave me a gigantic surge of self-confidence and increased my self-esteem.

If someone told me I was losing weight, it would send me into an eating binge so I could hear myself telling me I looked bigger.

I dreaded being sick because that meant I couldn't eat and thus would lose weight. I still dread being sick to this day for the same reason. The gallons of milk and boxes of cookies eventually gave me lactose intolerance and a 38-inch waistline.

But I didn't care because I was big. I was powerful. I didn't feel like a child anymore. I was, and still am somewhat, a grown man living with a child's view of the world.

As a child we are constantly seeking positive feedback and approval from adults around us. Some of us carry this natural attitude into our adult life.

We are always thinking about how others view us or whether we are liked.

How does this relate to body image? If our inner child is not healed, it will cry for attention and demand approval. It lives in a world of self-centrism. It's all about me.

How am I looking? Do you envy the way I look? Why aren't you complimenting me on my physique? Somehow I have to heal my inner child of the lack of acceptance and approval I didn't receive which has now surfaced in how I view my body and my unhealthy, obsession with feeling "like a grown-up".

I constantly remind my inner child that he's OK. He's safe and protected and to let myself drop my child-like view of the world in general.

The process is slow but it's improving. Certain thoughts are fading away. My inner child has been trying to protect me for a long time.

It's done a very good job. It, like the rest of us, wants to be accepted and loved. If you change your thoughts, you change your perception of reality."

I thanked my friend for sharing his deep feelings and thoughts.

Let's find comfort in knowing when looking at ourselves in a mirror asking, "Mirror, mirror on the wall, who's the fairest of them all?" that God's answer is He loves us just the way we are.

Who will be next?

Several years ago I attended a celebration of life honoring a fallen high school buddy who got called home at a too-young age of 51 years.

His father and older brother arranged a get-together celebration inviting those who knew him. The celebration included good food, drink and conversation.

I was excited about attending this long-overdue opportunity to mingle and engage in middle-aged man small talk with my former neighborhood and school friends.

I looked forward to catching up on what we had done since our youthful yesteryear high school days from long ago.

It's a shame, I thought, it took a funeral for old high school buddies from 95824 getting together and enjoying each others' company.

Some of my buddies were sporting bulging middle-aged man bellies while others sported gray, white or no hair.

One old friend had a body posture reminding me of an old rodeo cowboy who had been bucked off a rodeo bull one time too many.

"What do they think when looking at me?" I thought to myself.

What I discovered is while bellies may bulge, hair may turn gray or fall out, and body posture may lack youthful uprightness, the look in our eyes generally remains the same.

That turned out to be a fail-safe clue helping me identify my buddies because some of them were difficult to identify on first pass.

Among this crowd of old high school buddies were many sporting moustaches and a hair-combed-back style. Both of these were clues we're all middle-age men from the same time era.

While enjoying everyone's company, I repeatedly asked out, "Why does it take a funeral to get us together?"

And in the same breath and privately while reflecting on the life of my deceased high school buddy, I asked myself the question "Who will be next?"

Nothing I can do about it

Several years ago, the passing of my karate Sensei put me in touch with many people who I had not seen in a long time.

As I've reflected before, why does it take a funeral to get us together?

One person I spoke to was someone about 10 to 15 years my senior. He's a karate dojo brother from a different mother with a lifetime of karate training and still at it.

"How have you been doing?" I asked him during a telephone conversation.

I chuckled and enjoyed his perspective-loaded simple answer. He replied, *"I'm doing well but getting older and there's nothing I can do about it."*

Out of the loop

Several years ago my wife and I attended a wedding reception for a young couple we know.

She's a beautiful young woman and he's a handsome young man. They're both young enough to be my daughter and son.

Their private reception was at a popular night club closed to the public that night. It's a place frequented by young and beautiful single people wanting to be seen dressed for evening attractiveness success. They're often searching for Mr. or Miss Wonderful.

My wife and I exchanged occasional small talk with others while sampling delicious and plentiful hors d'oeuvres served as the reception meal.

As the night lingered on, I eventually felt overwhelmed by the loud music and density of beautiful and young single people with alcoholic beverages in hand, engaging in nightclub mingling while hunting for their evening scores.

My wife felt the same. We weren't the only middle-aged people among this vibrant crowd but definitely in the minority.

This place was a loud auditory and visual showcase of predictable Friday and Saturday late night dancing and drinking.

I knew from my own yesteryear memories many people here would be waking up next morning with hangovers, headaches and empty wallets.

The images from high to low and left to right reminded me of my own yesteryear days of living for and frequenting the night club scene.

It didn't take long before we were exhausted and overwhelmed from the loud music and density of beautiful and young people.

The straw breaking our camel's back was when a cocktail server brought us a small glass of champagne for toasting the bride and groom.

Neither my wife or I enjoy champagne so we both glanced at each other with glass in hand looking like fish out of water with a "What are we suppose to do with it?" look on our faces.

About fifteen minutes before 9:00 p.m. we made a mutually-agreeable "business decision" it was time to leave for our "safe" home. We quietly and unassumingly exited out a side door.

As the door shut, a dark alley greeted us with a pleasant breeze of fresh air and nighttime quietness in sharp contrast to the oxygen-thin nightclub air and decibel-piercing noise.

We held hands walking to our car. Looking at my wife, I told her we're both out of the loop.

Sucker punched in a nightclub brawl

Of all things I regularly do rejuvenating me, sleeping is at the top of my list. I'm no different than others and sleep away about one quarter to one third of my life.

Most middle-aged men like me sleep more because we take an occasional power nap when nobody is looking.

Does a tired old me take more naps than a younger average Joe 6-pack character?

Quite frankly, I don't know but perhaps I do even though I really don't take many naps.

But every now and then, generally on a Sunday afternoon, I'll treat myself to a two-hour-plus power nap. Man does that feel great!

What I do know is many middle-aged men have problems with interrupted sleep at night. My wife tells me middle-aged women also have this problem.

With middle-aged men, it's a middle-of-the-night trip to the bathroom when our prostate calls.

Mine is like a housedog scratching on a door in the middle of night with a doggy toilet alert.

I'm not sure why middle-aged women have interrupted sleep but maybe it's because their husbands are snoring.

Or maybe it's their own snoring keeping them awake.

Most of the time, I don't have a problem with interrupted sleep. I'm grateful yet know this is subject to change.

I generally feel calm, relaxed and sleepy at the end of a day. This feeling reminds me of being a young child when the sandman arrived. It was a very pleasant feeling then just like now.

It's seductive with accompanying rapid-fire flurries of sighs and yawns eventually leading me to a sudden lights-out knockout for a ten-count. Imagine a boxer who has just been knocked out in a fight; that's me.

Or imagine an image of a drunken sailor on liberty who just got sucker punched in a nightclub brawl.

Something is better than nothing

I used to have an "all or nothing" mentality about my fitness training. If I couldn't complete my entire planned workout, I wouldn't do anything at all.

This training mindset didn't serve me well because I experienced "fitness erosion" during times of the year when I was very busy with work.

Then I discovered a new mentality called "something is better than nothing" and my fitness conditioning has been better ever since.

I no longer experience as much fitness erosion with this something is better than nothing mentality.

Some of my best workouts with this training mentality were completed in 15 minutes or less early in the morning, leaving me plenty of time for a long day of work.

I personally like early morning workouts because they make me feel energetic and help me have a highly-productive day.

I've also learned the value of early-afternoon workouts on days when my middle-aged man bones and muscles need more time to wake up.

What I've learned is it's all good if we just show up and do it because something is better than nothing.

Forever never made it back to the gym

One evening several years ago, I returned to the gym after a three-week timeout. I had just completed a much-needed rest and recovery fitness training sabbatical.

I arrived at the gym around 6:10 p.m. that evening. Since time was short, I did an easy, fast and safe whole-body workout.

The barbell weights I chose were light and the repetitions and sets I performed were moderate. I was done 20 minutes later when the clock struck 6:30 p.m.

Easy as this workout was, I was sure the following afternoon would greet my body with some familiar delayed-onset muscle soreness (DOMS).

Quite frankly, I was looking forward to it.

In a reflective moment when beginning my cool-down, I thought about how good it felt to have jumped back on my fitness training saddle.

Three weeks was a long time off, or at least that was my perception. I've always said, as a middle-aged man, I'm only good as my last workout.

My reflective cool-down ended pondering about out-of-shape and overweight men and women who at one time were fit and trim, took some time off for rest and recovery, and forever never made it back to the gym.

Give me a big head

So here I go continuing in my ongoing middle-aged man fitness dude journey.

My fitness training and dietary practices have changed several times during my journey.

They were in response to changing interests and subtle aging that are part of my gracefully-aging work of art in progress.

There are at least three things I've learned in my journey.

First, my fitness training methods and dietary practices have got to match my personality for a lifetime commitment to health and wellness.

Second, I'm a middle-aged man only good as my last workout.

Third, I am what I eat.

While not a slam-dunk guarantee of authentic health and wellness, I admit having a lean and muscular body pleases me.

But honestly, the only thing it really ever did for me was give me a big head.

For the rest of my life

Others have asked me and I also constantly ask myself about how to best judge whether I've had a good fitness workout.

In my fitness past, I've gone through great periods of diet and exercise intensity producing great results.

Now I realize – while my Father Nature clock continues to tick tock toward the end of my life – the value of what I do today is best measured by whether I'll be able to do it for the rest of my life.

In pursuit of gracefully aging

I'm selective about what I read; reading only what really interests me and ignoring everything else.

At this middle-aged man point in my life, I've taken an interest in literature popularly-described as "anti-aging."

Anti-aging is not a term I invented; others did and I don't like it.

You see, there's nothing anti about aging in my book. It's an activity of the highest order; something we all do breath by breath, second by second, minute by minute, hour by hour, day by day, and year by year.

To live is to age and to age is to die. It's all been figured out and there's nothing I can do to change it.

So what's the meaning of anti-aging? It depends on who you ask.

According to the American Academy of Anti-Aging Medicine, until recently, medicine has presumed there's little I can do to alter aging but new scientific data reveals otherwise.

Their website states anti-aging medicine is a wellness-oriented model of advanced clinical preventive medicine devoted to achieving demonstrable and objective results that beneficially impact the degenerative disease of aging.

What the heck does this mean?

Remember, I'm a middle-aged man meathead needing to be talked to in a way I can understand. I don't understand this gobbledygook.

I've learned anti-aging medicine is a field not recognized by established medical organizations, such as the American Board of American Specialties or the American Medical Association.

That's not a deal breaker for me since I've never been a fan of mainstream establishments.

Still, I don't like the term "anti-aging" for the reason stated above.

This anti-aging stuff, in my mind, falls under the umbrella of there's nothing new under the sun.

What's practiced now may in reality not be much different than efforts of Spanish explorer Ponce de Leon over 500 years ago in his futile search for the Fountain of Youth to cure his aging.

Every man who looks in a mirror sees a 16-year-old kid I constantly tell myself. I know I'm not alone in my thoughts.

So true is this my mindscape that it's easy to understand why I have such an interest in this anti-aging stuff.

Still, I don't like this "anti-aging" term and refuse to use it other than acknowledging it exists in fitness and medical literature.

For me, I prefer thinking my efforts in chasing fitness, health and wellness are all in pursuit of gracefully aging.

Diet and fitness affirmations from A to Z

One year in late December with a new year around the corner, I wrote my diet and fitness affirmations from A to Z to share with fellow middle-aged men and anyone else interested.

Allow me to share them with you.

A word of caution - I'm not a professional nutritionist or fitness trainer so please take what I share with a grain of salt and a pound of caution.

Also, you should consult your health care professional before embarking on any health and wellness program making sure it's appropriate for you.

A – Always train a little on scheduled fitness training days. Don't let your efforts be sabotaged by an "all or nothing" mentality because something is better than nothing.

B – Be on guard for family and friends not sharing your diet and fitness zeal because their misguided charity, perhaps loaded with envy, can sabotage your efforts.

C – Chance is not how diet and fitness improvements are made so make sure you have a written plan guiding your daily efforts.

D – Don't eat unless you're hungry. Break old habits of eating because the clock says it's a certain time or food is offered to you when you're not hungry. Don't be afraid to say "No thank you."

E – Eat your food slowly and make sure you "milkshakefy" it. What's that mean? Read **The Pierini DIET**, a free and easy-read PDF book I've written. Send me an e-mail and I'll send you a free copy.

F – Fuel your body with real food because it'll support the demands of your fitness training and aid in post-training recovery.

G – **Go** for a brisk walk as an alternative to watching television or spending time on the computer. You can always get back to your television or computer after taking your brisk walk.

H – **Have** fun chasing your diet and fitness goals and you'll increase the likelihood of success.

I – **Intensity** is your time-efficient friend so make sure your cardio sessions are short and intense rather than long, slow and steady. You should be bordering on breathlessness at the end of your cardio training.

J – **Jump** if you can now and then in your training. It's a great way to keep your cardio sessions short and intense.

K – **Kill** all negative thoughts periodically entering your mind that you can't achieve your diet and fitness goals. Find something else to be a failure about.

L – **Lift** heavy weights at least once, and preferably, twice a week following a progressive resistance training program.

Use good form and seek out instruction making sure you're performing all lifts correctly and safely.

M – Monitor your bodyweight, diet and fitness training efforts by maintaining a journal. Record all details in your journal. Depending on your dietary discipline, consider using a daily food journal. It'll help you be aware of what you're eating and foster your rigorous honesty.

N – Never tell yourself you can't do it because you can – if you want it bad enough.

O – Opportunities for eating healthy and exercising are always present, even when you're away on a business trip or vacation. Be creative and do something. Don't worry about people looking at you – let them.

P – Pushups, pullups and other bodyweight-only exercises should be part of your fitness training program because fitness training variety is the results-producing spice of life.

Q – Question all you read and are told about diet and fitness from the *"experts."*

Follow money and motives making sure their advice passes your *"smell test."*

R – Rest and recovery are your friends after a hard fitness training session. Train hard and then make sure you have quality rest and recovery on non-training days.

S – Sitting is something you do when eating, visiting with friends and working if you sit for a living. While exercising, don't lay when you can sit but don't sit when you can stand.

T – Timed workouts are great particularly during short and intense cardio sessions. Use a stop watch occasionally and time your efforts. It'll help you do a better job of measuring your fitness improvement.

U – Umbrellas can be used when taking a brisk walk on a rainy day rather than talking yourself out of doing so because it's raining. Make sure you have one in you fitness training tool box.

V – Victims of crimes sometimes put themselves in harm's way. Don't be a victim of diet and fitness failure crime by putting yourself in harm's way with environments and people not safe for you.

W – Warm-up your body with flexibility drills and gradually elevate your heart rate before beginning the tough part of your fitness training.

X – X-treme and unrealistic diet and fitness goals should be avoided. Reasonably demanding and achievable goals will serve you better.

Y – Yearn for the day when you're closer to achieving your diet and fitness goals for that's today.

Z – Zeal will serve you well in your lifelong diet and fitness journey. Make sure you're always carrying some with you.

There you have it folks – my diet and fitness affirmations from A to Z.

Only 50 words

My middle-aged man written reflections are probably, on average, about 500 words. Some people have told me my writings tend to be too wordy.

Lately, I've toyed with an idea of shorter written reflections so this one is an attempt to see what one looks like with only 50 words.

Middle-aged man health and wellness exam

Since I pay my own health insurance, I've chosen a high-deductible plan lowering my health insurance premium cost.

Lower monthly premiums save me money but this policy has a higher annual deductible. This means I use more of my own money for medical expenses before the insurance policy starts paying. In healthy years, it may not pay anything.

I'm gambling the premium savings will be more than my annual out-of-pocket costs.

Thus far, this policy has served me well. It has made me a better consumer of health care motivating me to have greater ownership of my health and wellness.

As a result of this motivation, I've created a self-administered exam for periodically self-assessing my middle-aged man health and wellness.

I've had fun sharing this exam with other middle-aged men and would like sharing it with you.

First of all, know I'm not a health care professional so take what I say with a grain of salt, pound of caution and good old-fashioned belly laugh.

This self-exam consists of five questions all of which you answer yes or no. You need at least four yes answers to pass.

Passing the exam means I have good middle-aged man health and wellness and, therefore, don't need to go to a doctor.

Again, I'm not a health care professional so take ownership of your middle-aged man health and wellness deciding if you should consult with your health care professional before taking this self-examination.

So here's the exam; again answer each question with a yes or no answer. "It depends" is not an acceptable answer.

First, at the end of a day, do you remember what you had for breakfast?

Second, can you walk up a single-story flight of stairs without being winded when getting to the top?

Third, can you bend over and pick up something off the floor without throwing out your back or ripping the seat of your pants?

Fourth, can you get through a whole day without crapping your pants?

At this point, if you're jumping with joy because you've answered yes to these four questions, good for you because you've passed the exam regardless of whether you answer yes to the fifth and final question for a perfect score.

Drum roll please – fifth, can you piss over a six foot fence?

Yikes! That's a tough one.

Many middle-aged men I've shared this exam with laugh hard when asked this final question.

Some answer yes but most answer no. I always tell those who answer no but who answered yes to the other four questions:

> *"No problem, buy a trampoline. Congratulations, you've passed the exam and are a middle-aged man specimen of good health and wellness."*

So there you have it my friends, my middle-aged man health and wellness exam.

Like a splash of Old Spice

I once read a news article about a research project catching my attention. It reported old people do smell, but not badly.

This article interested me because, as a middle-aged man, I know old man land will soon be my landscape and mindscape.

A group of purported scientists with nothing better to do conducted a study where participants were given "whiffs" from pieces of pads worn under armpits of young, middle-aged and elderly people for five consecutive nights.

Researchers discovered study participants were able to reliably distinguish body odors of the elderly, who were 75 years and older.

May this middle-aged man bellow a sigh of relief since he's not 75 years or older?

Does this also answer a private question of "Grandpa, do you really stink?"

No, because participants rated middle-aged man body odor the worst and strongest.

"Those are fighting words!" shouts this middle-aged man.

As a self-proclaimed ambassador and tireless advocate of middle-aged men of the world, I must defend my brothers from different mothers from this research nonsense.

I've always been slightly skeptical of scientific research knowing its design and findings can be skewed by who funds it.

Obviously this research was funded by women since the study found odor from women of all ages as less intense than men, and closer to neutral smelling for young and middle-aged people.

Do I hear the sound of an Avon lady calling?

Well this middle-aged man isn't buying any of this scientific research nonsense.

I've said it time and time again – every man who looks in a mirror sees a 16-year-old kid.

I also believe this from the bottom of my heart - this middle-aged man will always smell nice like a splash of Old Spice.

I miss my Gangee

Every October 26th, I think about my dear and departed maternal grandmother who I knew as and called *Gangee*. She was born on October 26, 1900.

I was so close to her that, as a U.S. Army soldier stationed in the Republic of Korea, my sergeant approved a 30-day emergency leave request in March 1975 so I could fly home and be with her when she was critically ill.

I clearly remember a long 14-hour flight home to California wondering my entire trip how she was doing and whether she was still alive.

I also remember first words uttered upon arriving of "How is she?" and my uncle's answer she had passed away.

I immediately broke into tears. Later that night, I cried my guts out in a torrential storm of tears while tossing and turning in bed wanting to believe it was just a bad dream.

Without a doubt, I was her favorite grandchild; there's always one who has that honor and, with her, it was me.

As a young boy, I spent lots of time visiting her and together we watched her favorite programs on her black and white television set.

She enjoyed watching western series like Bonanza and Gunsmoke. She also enjoyed wholesome variety shows like the Perry Como Show, Ed Sullivan Show and Lawrence Welk Show.

All her grandchildren knew her as Gangee. It was a name I gave her according to my Dad. Gangee was my baby-version of a failed attempt calling her grandma.

Every year in October on her birthday, I visit her grave at the cemetery praying and reflecting about how much I miss my Gangee.

Your son eternally

The following is a poem my father wrote to his father. I share it as a dedication to both of them. They've both gone home to their Heavenly Father for their eternal rest.

To Dad

Damn it dad, why did you go?
You told me one-hundred, and I believed you,

And all that went in to making you,
But you "tripped" before your time.

I remember the day, when I misbehaved,

And you placed your strong hand on my shoulder.

I may have wept.

But you are gone now, but not the hand,
Which, on this cold night, I kneel to kiss.

Eddie, your son, eternally

Buona Pasqua 2013

I shared the following with my Dad when spending Easter Sunday 2013 with him. He was dying a painful and slow death from a rare form of cancer.

He died less than two months later on May 24, 2013.

Caro Padre,

Thank you for giving me life, my Catholic faith, for correcting me when I did wrong and praising me when I did right, for inspiring me to develop a personal sense of self worth and to stick up for myself.

Thank you for cultivating in me a joy of health and wellness and a love for the iron barbell.

Thank you for all those great conversations and sharing our Pierini Family history that I promise I'll pass on to the next generation.

Thank you for spending this Easter Sunday 2013 with me and giving me another wonderful day of being your son.

All these treasures you've given me have made me a "rich man."

"Ti amo molto; la pace del Signore sia sempre con te" - Eddie

Happy Birthday Dear Elizabeth

I wrote this birthday poem for my wife on September 8, 2013:

Today's your birthday, let's celebrate your life, and enjoy today my sweet loving wife;

The crosses you've carried in recent past, with prayers to God they will not last;

Many love you in ways you'll never know, sometimes though it might not show;

A new decade of life you're about to live, with many joys you'll receive and give;

In the name of the Father, Son and Holy Ghost, your beauty and goodness is what I love most;

I pray to God from the bottom of my heart, the rest of your life we'll never be apart;

Happy birthday and know this my dear wife, God will give you many blessings for the rest of your life.

Happy Birthday Dear Elizabeth.

Dime a dozen

My pursuit of gracefully aging is always fun, sometimes challenging, and full of blessings but also with occasional heavy crosses to carry.

We all carry a cross at some point in our lives and during those times when mine seem heaviest, I find relief knowing my crosses are no greater than what God has determined I'm capable of carrying.

My gracefully aging journey has given me much self-discovery and personal maturity, and sage wisdom from trying my very best of living a good and honest life.

This feel-good feeling I have can't be matched from any feelings I have of being a "big shot" in circles I frequent on a regular basis, satisfaction of my professional career and education, or material belongings and high-society contacts I "own" fitting me into, or excluding me from, a certain socio-economic pecking order of society.

Let me share something from the bottom of my mind, body and soul — *"Humble pie tastes a whole lot better than ego cake!"*

I don't know about you but my self-realization is despite how good and great I may think I am, I'm not alone but rather in company of many who are as good and great and even greater than me.

I find it very humbling to remind myself as I ponder in a moment of bliss, and an everlasting awakening of who I am and who I want to be, that I'm nothing more than a dime a dozen.

My final 100 things

I once read a news article about a middle-aged man medical doctor living his last days in the final stages of a neurological disorder known as Lou Gehrig's disease.

This afflicted doctor shared how he found himself unable to lift his arms above his head so he had to give up basketball and golf, and how he cut short his medical career when he grew too tired to get through a work day.

He quit singing when forming words became too difficult. The article shared how this 55-year young middle-aged man had been contemplating how many more losses he could endure before his life was no longer worth living.

What attracted me to this article were two things.

First, he was my physician many years ago and I clearly remember a disagreement with him and giving him a piece of my mind.

Second, as a card-carrying 100 percent Roman Catholic, I found something this dying doctor shared aligning with my faith and belief - life ends only when God and nobody else decides.

He shared how he was against euthanasia and assisted suicide.

He still believed in the Hippocratic Oath he learned in medical school pledging doctors will give no deadly medicine nor suggest any such counsel.

My food for thought in this article was his sharing how he maintained a mental list of things most important to him like kissing his wife, taking vacations, and enjoying food.

He shared how he would be ready to die when he had lost "enough things that matter."

He called his approach "100 things."

When I finished reading this article, I promised myself I would include my former doctor and his family in my prayers and thoughts while he enjoyed his final days.

Also, in private reflection, I thanked my former doctor and fellow middle-aged man for cultivating in me a desire to define my final 100 things.

It was fun while it lasted

Gracefully aging is not always a smooth trip for me and in its journey I sometimes hit a rough spot on the road leaving my car of life with a few dings.

That's been my recent discovery after spending time this past year looking in a mirror.

These views are not familiar front-facing ones that never disappoint me and always please me with illusory images in my mind's eye of my 16-year-old kid alter ego.

Instead, they're rear and top views using a hand-held mirror with my backside facing a larger bathroom mirror.

And what am I seeing from these vantage points?

I'm seeing a middle-aged man who's losing hair on top of his head.

It's not very visible to most but nonetheless it's my biological commotion in motion.

I wouldn't go so far to say I'm going bald; that's too drastic of a statement yet, but it's fair to say – and read my lips – "My hair is thinning and I'm losing hair."

"Yikes!" yells this distressed middle-aged man.

It wasn't long ago I was a newbie middle-aged man sporting a mullet badge of honor just for kicks.

While never topically-endowed like the late great musician Freddy Fender by any stretch of my imagination, I wore an eccentric mullet royal crown covering my head and draping my neck. It soothed my rebel in remission soul giving me much middle-aged man satisfaction.

But that was then and this is now and, despite my best efforts being in denial and talking myself out of what's happening, I must confess my hair is thinning and I'm losing my hair. To where will this discovery lead me?

Will I be the next Yul Bryner, ready for a leading actor role in a 21st century remake of "The King and I"? Or maybe I'll qualify working as a 21st century version of the television ad character known as "Mr. Clean."

The opportunities are endless proving there are blessings to be found in crosses I carry.

This whole experience may not be like stepping on dog poop but rather finding my next diamond in the rough.

The ball is in my court and it's up to me to make the best of it.

I truly believe in darkness of a night my stars will shine the brightest.

I'm ready to go with the flow, to be content with the biological deck of cards God has dealt me, and to find goodness and gratefulness in all other good things going on in my health and wellness journey.

The best way to sum up my thoughts about a disappearing thick head of hair is to say it was fun while it lasted.

They're good and gone

Time can be classified into three time buckets: past, present and future. My good times can likewise be classified as: good old days, good now days and good days to come.

You know your good old days well like just like me and we both spend countless hours telling countless stories about them.

Some of my pleasant good old days memories are about attending high school, buying and driving my first car, serving as a soldier in the U.S. Army, attending college, courting and marrying my wife and being a father to my little daughter and son.

I probably enjoy listening to other people's good old day stories more than telling my own. Listening to my father's stories during the last couple years of his life, for example, provided me much joy. They also added to my own inventory of good old day stories.

Good now days are what I'm presently living. Sometimes, though, the goodness of them gets blurred by crosses I carry in my rest-of-life journey.

Like watching my father die a horrific and painful death, struggling to meet special needs of a sick wife, and little aches and pains shouting at me inside my middle-aged man body.

There are others but, when they surface and control my now being, I pretend they don't exist by replacing them with pleasant thoughts from my good old days or good days to come.

The good days to come, for me, seem something I pondered about more when a young college student. They were a "great high" particularly when a safe distance from what was then my now.

Like, for example, when I was a sophomore in college and my blue sky peaches and cream good days to come were a couple years away from being put to reality tests.

Pleasant thoughts about my good days to come were plentiful then and greatly contributed to euphoria I regularly experienced.

My thoughts about living the golden years of my life, I suppose, should provide a similar euphoria but thus far this hasn't been my case.

Time will eventually tell and one day when sitting in a rocking chair during the 11th hour of my life watching time go by, I may have a different perspective than now.

So which of these good times is my favorite? This is a question I recently asked myself. After some private reflection, I'm not sure.

There's a natural attraction I have for my good old days. I believe the older I get the more this natural attraction will grow.

Maybe that's why I enjoy listening to older people's stories about their good old days. They seem to share their stories better than I do and listening to them is more enjoyable than telling my own.

However, just like the "The devil is in the details." expression, my pleasant yesteryear memories of my good old days may really be "deceptive in their distance."

This deception may undermine the goodness of both my good now days and my, hopefully, good days to come.

A friend's perspective may have said it best when he recently shared good old days are good because they're good and gone.

Who are you?

It's no well-kept secret - my daily encounters with a bathroom mirror.

This daily morning ritual has been the subject of several of my favorite middle-aged man written reflections and discussions with anyone giving me a courtesy of their ears.

Without a doubt, my favorite one-liner reflection is that every man who looks in a mirror sees a 16-year-old kid.

For those who take me too seriously, know I'm not alone.

The late great radio and television comedian Jack Benny was known for his public character of being age 39 years regardless of how old he really was.

The late great Spanish artist Pablo Picasso once said at age 76 years, *"Everyone is the age he has decided on, and I have decided to remain 30."*

I may be overstepping my boundaries including myself among these famous people.

But excluding me doesn't leave me alone because there are many other middle-aged men and women adoring and marveling their mirror image reflecting back at them from their Fountain of Youth bathroom mirrors.

Do I suffer from narcissism, megalomania, egocentrism or some other personality disorder made up by those characters known as psychologists who take joy in classifying crazy people like me into well-described buckets of personality disorders and mental illness?

I wonder if I'm a modern-day Narcissus – a Greek mythology character renowned for his beauty - attracted to a pool where I see my own reflection in water and fall in love with it.

Heck no in my most private thoughts but that'll never keep me from having fun fooling all those naïve enough to take me seriously.

At this point in my life, there's no way I see a 16-year-old kid when looking in a mirror.

Rather, these daily morning encounters have me looking at my mirror image and asking a very tough question - "Who are you?"

A middle-aged man named Pierini

Edward Joseph (Ed) Pierini, Jr. is a fourth-generation native of Sacramento, California where he resides with Elizabeth, his wife of 35 years. They have two adult children who hopefully will one day be their middle-aged daughter and son.

A high school dropout who joined the U.S. Army in his senior year, Ed later redeemed himself by earning two university degrees and becoming a Certified Public Accountant (CPA). He's now a CPA in private practice.

Ed calls himself an ambassador of middle-aged men around the world. He enjoys coaching and mentoring other middle-aged men seeking to live a good and honest life.

He'd like your feedback about his book and he'll do his very best to answer any questions you have.

You may contact him via e-mail at **pierinifitness@gmail.com**.